CONTENTS

INTRODUCTION

*The Artistry of 5-
Ingredient Cuisine*

In the realm of culinary arts, the concept of 5-ingredient cuisine stands as an epitome of simplicity and creativity. Embracing this approach to cooking involves crafting flavorful, satisfying dishes using only a handful of key components. The restriction to five ingredients necessitates an ingenious selection of elements, encouraging a focus on quality, balance, and innovation. It's a canvas where chefs and home cooks alike can unleash their creativity, relying on the essence of ingredients to elevate flavors and textures.

Elements of 5-Ingredient Mastery

1. **Ingredient Selection**: The essence of 5-ingredient cuisine lies in the careful curation of elements. Each ingredient must play a pivotal role, harmonizing with others to create a symphony of flavors. The selection process involves not only choosing top-quality items but also considering their versatility. A handful of ingredients must

possess the potential to manifest diverse tastes and textures, allowing for multifaceted dishes.

2. **Balance and Harmony**: Achieving equilibrium among the selected ingredients is crucial. It's about understanding their inherent qualities—tanginess, sweetness, bitterness, umami—and blending them in a way that each element complements the others. This balance amplifies the overall taste, making the dish greater than the sum of its parts.

3. **Technique and Innovation**: Limited ingredients breed innovation. Chefs and cooks explore various techniques—grilling, roasting, braising, etc.—to bring out the best in each component. Experimentation becomes key, leading to unconventional pairings and methods that unlock unexpected flavors and textures.

4. **Presentation and Aesthetics**: Simplicity doesn't mean compromising aesthetics. The visual appeal of a dish in 5-ingredient cuisine is essential. Chefs focus on presentation techniques that highlight the beauty of the ingredients, making the dish inviting and appetizing.

Unlocking Culinary Creativity with Five Ingredients

The beauty of this minimalist approach to cooking lies in its democratization of gourmet meals. It empowers both seasoned chefs and novice cooks to create impressive dishes with limited resources. It promotes innovation, challenges the traditional norms of cooking, and encourages exploration of different cuisines and flavors.

Accessibility and Health Benefits

Beyond its creative potential, 5-ingredient cuisine offers accessibility and health benefits. By simplifying recipes and reducing the number of ingredients, it becomes more approachable for individuals with limited cooking experience or access to a variety of ingredients. Moreover, this approach often leads to healthier meals, as it encourages the use of fresh, whole foods in their natural state, minimizing reliance on processed or pre-packaged items.

Purpose and Scope of this Ebook

This Ebook is designed as a comprehensive guide to delve into the world of 5-ingredient cuisine. It aims to equip readers with the knowledge, skills, and inspiration to embrace the artistry of minimalist cooking. Through a collection of recipes, cooking techniques, and insights from culinary experts, this Ebook endeavors to empower individuals to create delightful, restaurant-worthy dishes using only five key ingredients.

Objectives of the Ebook

1. **Education and Guidance**: The primary goal is to educate readers about the fundamentals of 5-ingredient cuisine. It provides insights into ingredient selection, flavor pairing, cooking techniques, and the principles of achieving balance and harmony in dishes.

2. **Inspiration and Creativity**: The Ebook serves as a source of inspiration, sparking creativity in the kitchen. It offers a variety of recipes across different cuisines, encouraging experimentation and innovation while maintaining simplicity.

3. **Empowerment and Accessibility**: By simplifying

complex cooking methods and focusing on a minimal ingredient list, this Ebook aims to empower individuals of all skill levels to create impressive meals. It promotes accessibility to gourmet-style cooking without the need for a vast array of ingredients or advanced culinary expertise.

4. **Health and Well-being**: Another significant aspect is promoting healthier eating habits. The Ebook emphasizes the use of fresh, wholesome ingredients, thereby advocating for a more nutritious approach to cooking and eating.

Empowering Readers through Minimalist Cooking

Minimalist cooking extends beyond the reduction of ingredients; it's a philosophy that embodies simplicity, creativity, and mindfulness in the culinary process. By embracing minimalism, cooks can focus on the essentials, fostering a deeper connection with the ingredients and the cooking experience itself.

Benefits of Minimalist Cooking

1. **Streamlined Process**: Simplifying the ingredient list streamlines the cooking process, making it less intimidating and time-consuming. This approach encourages efficiency in meal preparation.

2. **Enhanced Flavor Appreciation**: By using fewer ingredients, the nuances of flavors are highlighted, allowing individuals to truly appreciate and savor each component in a dish.

3. **Reduced Food Waste**: A focus on minimalism often leads to more conscientious ingredient

usage, reducing food waste. This aligns with sustainability goals by advocating for mindful consumption.

4. **Cultivation of Creativity**: Limitations breed creativity. Minimalist cooking challenges individuals to think outside the box, fostering culinary innovation and personal expression in the kitchen.

5. **Promotion of Mindful Eating**: Through a minimalist approach, individuals are encouraged to be more mindful of what they consume, leading to a greater appreciation for food and its impact on overall well-being.

EMBRACING THE ESSENCE OF 5-INGREDIENT RECIPES

Defining the Concept of 5-Ingredient Cooking

The concept of 5-ingredient cooking revolves around the art of creating delicious and satisfying meals using a minimal number of ingredients. Its essence lies in simplicity, focusing on quality ingredients and allowing their flavors to shine without complex recipes or extensive preparation. The idea is not merely about counting ingredients but rather embracing simplicity and efficiency in the kitchen.

1. Emphasis on Simplicity: 5-ingredient cooking embodies the ethos of simplicity. By limiting the ingredient count, it encourages cooks to focus on the quality of each component. The limited number of ingredients challenges creativity while making the cooking process more manageable.

2. Quality Over Quantity: This concept prioritizes the quality of ingredients over quantity. Each ingredient chosen plays a crucial role in flavor and texture, ensuring that every element contributes significantly to the dish's overall taste profile.

3. Streamlined Preparation: With fewer ingredients, the cooking process becomes more streamlined. It reduces the time spent on chopping, prepping, and cooking, making it an ideal approach for busy individuals seeking homemade meals without sacrificing taste or nutrition.

4. Flexibility and Adaptability: Despite the limitation on the number of ingredients, 5-ingredient cooking allows for versatility. Ingredients can be substituted or varied to suit dietary preferences, making it accessible for different dietary needs, whether vegan, gluten-free, or others.

Benefits and Value Proposition

The practice of 5-ingredient cooking offers numerous benefits and a compelling value proposition for both amateur and seasoned cooks.

1. Time Efficiency: One of the primary advantages is time efficiency. With fewer ingredients and simplified cooking processes, meals can be prepared swiftly, making it an appealing option for individuals with busy schedules.

2. Cost-Effectiveness: Another notable benefit is its cost-effectiveness. By using a limited number of ingredients, one can reduce grocery expenses while minimizing food wastage. This approach allows individuals to make the most of what they have without excessive spending.

3. Enhanced Focus on Flavor and Ingredients: The limited ingredient list encourages heightened focus on the flavors and characteristics of each component. This results in dishes that highlight the natural taste of the ingredients, leading to a more enjoyable culinary experience.

4. Minimalistic Approach to Cooking: 5-ingredient cooking promotes a minimalist approach to cooking, simplifying the meal preparation process. This appeals to individuals seeking simplicity in their lives, fostering a less cluttered and more organized cooking experience.

5. Healthier Eating Habits: The simplicity of this cooking style often leads to healthier eating habits. By relying on a smaller number of ingredients, individuals are inclined to use fresh and wholesome options, contributing to a more nutritious diet.

Strategies for Crafting Flavorful Minimalist Dishes

Creating flavorful dishes with a minimal number of ingredients requires strategic planning and a keen understanding of how different components interact to elevate taste profiles.

1. Choose Flavorful Ingredients: Opt for ingredients that pack a punch in terms of flavor. Ingredients like fresh herbs, spices, citrus zest, aged cheeses, and high-quality oils can enhance the taste of the dish without needing a multitude of components.

2. Layering Flavors: Utilize cooking techniques like sautéing, roasting, or caramelizing to bring out the natural sweetness or depth of flavors in the ingredients. Layering flavors by adding ingredients at different stages of cooking can amplify taste complexity.

3. Balance and Contrast: Achieve a balanced flavor profile by incorporating contrasting elements such as sweet and savory, acidic and creamy, or spicy and mild. This contrast adds depth and excitement to the dish.

4. **Experimentation and Creativity:** Encourage experimentation and creativity in the kitchen. Don't be afraid to try unconventional ingredient pairings or cooking methods. Sometimes, the most unexpected combinations result in extraordinary flavors.

5. Focus on Texture: Texture plays a vital role in the enjoyment of a dish. Incorporate ingredients with varying textures - crunchy, creamy, chewy, or crispy - to add dimension and interest to the meal.

NAVIGATING FLAVOR HARMONY WITH FEW INGREDIENTS

*Navigating Flavor Harmony
with Few Ingredients*

When it comes to creating culinary wonders with limited ingredients, mastering flavor harmony is essential. Whether it's a dish composed of a handful of components or a minimalist approach to cooking, understanding how flavors interact and complement each other is key.

Understanding Basic Flavor Profiles: At the heart of flavor harmony lies the understanding of basic flavor profiles: sweet, salty, sour, bitter, and umami. Each taste plays a pivotal role in creating a balanced dish. For instance, when combining few ingredients, using a touch of sweetness to offset bitterness or adding acidity to cut through richness can transform the overall taste profile.

Embracing Contrast and Complement: One approach to achieving flavor harmony with few ingredients is by embracing both contrast and complement. Contrast allows for dynamic flavors to stand out, while complement ensures a cohesive blend. For instance, pairing the richness of roasted vegetables with a tangy vinaigrette or balancing the heat of spicy ingredients with cooling elements like yogurt or cucumber offers a delightful contrast.

Utilizing Aromatics and Herbs: Aromatics and herbs wield an incredible power to elevate simple dishes. Even with a minimal ingredient list, incorporating fresh herbs like basil, cilantro, or mint can impart layers of complexity. Their aromatic qualities can add depth and nuance, transforming a plain dish into a vibrant culinary experience.

Exploring Ethnic Flavor Combinations: Exploring different ethnic cuisines provides a treasure trove of flavor combinations. For example, the simplicity of Italian cuisine often revolves around a few key ingredients, showcasing how ingredients like tomatoes, basil, and olive oil can work harmoniously together. Similarly, Asian cuisines frequently utilize soy sauce, ginger, garlic, and sesame oil to create intricate yet balanced flavors.

Balancing Tastes and Textures

Achieving a harmonious balance between tastes and textures in a dish is an art form. While taste refers to the flavors perceived on the palate, textures contribute to the overall sensory experience. Mastering this interplay enhances the enjoyment of a dish, especially when working with limited ingredients.

Play of Textures: Incorporating various textures, such as crispy, creamy, chewy, or crunchy, adds dimension to a dish. For instance, pairing a tender protein with a crispy element, like a crunchy crust or roasted nuts, can elevate the eating experience by providing a delightful contrast in textures.

Taste Balance: Balancing tastes within the dish ensures that no single flavor overwhelms the palate. Achieving this balance involves adjusting the proportions of sweet, salty, sour, bitter, and umami tastes. For instance, a dish containing a salty component can be complemented with a touch of sweetness to achieve a more harmonious overall taste profile.

Layering Flavors: Layering flavors involves building complexity by adding ingredients in stages throughout the cooking process. For instance, starting a dish with a base of caramelized onions, then gradually adding garlic, herbs, spices, and finally finishing with a splash of acidity can create a depth of flavor even with limited ingredients.

Contrasting Textures with Taste: Combining contrasting textures with tastes can create an intriguing dining experience. Pairing a tangy sauce with a smooth and velvety puree or serving a spicy dish with a cooling element not only balances tastes but also contrasts textures, enhancing the overall enjoyment of the meal.

Highlighting Ingredients for Optimal Flavor Impact

Making the most of limited ingredients involves maximizing the flavors of each component. Highlighting key ingredients can create a focal point, allowing their flavors to shine through and create a memorable dining experience.

Ingredient Quality: The quality of ingredients plays a crucial role in flavor impact. Opting for fresh, seasonal produce or high-quality proteins can significantly enhance the overall taste of a dish. Freshness intensifies flavors and elevates the dining experience, even with minimal ingredients.

Focus on Technique: Mastering cooking techniques like caramelization, searing, roasting, or braising can amplify the flavors of ingredients. These techniques unlock hidden depths within ingredients, intensifying their natural flavors and textures.

Minimalist Approach: Embracing a minimalist approach allows each ingredient to take center stage. For instance, a simple caprese salad with fresh tomatoes, mozzarella, basil, and a drizzle of olive oil emphasizes the vibrant flavors of the ingredients without overwhelming the palate.

Synergy of Ingredients: Identifying the synergy between ingredients helps in showcasing their best attributes. Understanding which flavors complement or enhance each other allows for thoughtful pairing, ensuring that each ingredient contributes positively to the overall dish.

Case Studies and Flavor Pairing Experiments

Exploring case studies and conducting flavor pairing experiments offer valuable insights into creating flavorful dishes with limited ingredients. These experiments provide a platform for understanding how different flavors interact and complement each other.

Case Studies in Cuisine: Studying renowned dishes from various cuisines that utilize minimal ingredients can offer inspiration and insights. Analyzing classics like bruschetta, ratatouille, or a classic caprese salad can reveal the artistry behind combining a few key ingredients to create memorable dishes.

Experimental Pairings: Conducting flavor pairing experiments allows for a deeper understanding of ingredient interactions. For instance, experimenting with different herbs, spices, acids, and fats to see how they enhance or alter the flavors of a dish can lead to surprising and innovative combinations.

Sensory Evaluation: Employing sensory evaluation techniques, such as taste-testing panels or blind tastings, can help in understanding how different flavor combinations are perceived by individuals. This approach aids in refining and perfecting flavor harmonies with limited ingredients.

Innovative Fusion: Experimenting with fusion cuisine by combining elements from different culinary traditions can lead to innovative flavor profiles. The amalgamation of diverse ingredients opens up new possibilities for creating exciting and unexpected taste experiences.

STREAMLINING CULINARY CREATIONS: TIME-SAVING TECHNIQUES

Effective Meal Planning Strategies in 5 Ingredients

Meal planning can be a time-consuming task, but with strategic approaches focusing on minimal ingredients, it can become simpler and more efficient. To begin with, consider the following key points:

1. **Ingredient Selection**: Opt for versatile ingredients that can be used in multiple dishes. Staples like chicken breast, rice, beans, eggs, and a variety of vegetables serve as a great foundation.

2. **Diversify Flavors**: Despite the limitation of ingredients, aim to include a range of flavors by utilizing different spices, herbs, or sauces. This can significantly enhance the taste of the meals.

3. **Preparation Efficiency**: Plan meals that require minimal preparation time. Choose recipes that involve straightforward cooking methods such as stir-frying, roasting, or simple assembling.

Efficient meal planning within the constraint of five ingredients involves a blend of creativity and practicality. One effective strategy is to **utilize leftovers creatively**. For instance, grilled chicken from one meal can be repurposed into a salad or sandwich the next day, saving time and reducing waste.

Quick Prep and Cooking Hacks

In today's fast-paced lifestyle, quick prep and cooking hacks are invaluable. Here are some **noteworthy points to consider**:

1. **Prep in Batches**: Spend a portion of your day or week prepping ingredients in advance. Wash and chop vegetables, marinate proteins, or cook a large batch of grains, allowing for quick assembly during mealtime.

2. **One-Pot Wonders**: Opt for recipes that involve minimal cleanup by cooking everything in a single pot or pan. Dishes like stir-fries, casseroles, or sheet pan meals simplify both cooking and cleaning processes.

3. **Use Kitchen Gadgets**: Employ time-saving kitchen gadgets such as pressure cookers, slow cookers, or air fryers. These devices significantly

reduce cooking time while retaining flavors and nutrients.

Quick cooking hacks often revolve around optimizing time and effort. **The integration of shortcuts and efficient cooking techniques** allows individuals to prepare delicious meals without spending excessive time in the kitchen.

Maximizing Flavor with Minimal Effort

Enhancing flavor while minimizing effort is a challenge, but it's achievable with strategic choices. **Consider the following points to maximize flavor with minimal effort**:

1. **Layering Flavors**: Utilize ingredients that pack a punch in flavor, such as garlic, ginger, citrus zest, or chili flakes. Layering these elements enhances the taste profile without adding more ingredients.

2. **Quality Ingredients**: Invest in high-quality spices, herbs, and condiments. Even with a limited number of ingredients, using fresh and flavorful components can significantly elevate the dish.

3. **Balancing Flavors**: Aim for a balance of flavors— sweet, salty, sour, bitter, and umami—within the dish. This harmony creates depth and richness, enhancing the overall taste.

Efficiency in maximizing flavor often revolves around understanding the synergy between different ingredients and how they interact to create a well-rounded taste experience.

EXPLORING GLOBAL FLAVORS IN 5 INGREDIENTS

Adapting International Cuisines

Adapting international cuisines while staying true to their essence requires a delicate balance between respecting traditions and allowing for innovative twists. 1. Research and Understanding: Before adapting a cuisine, deep dive into its core components, cooking techniques, and the philosophy behind it. Understanding the soul of the cuisine helps in retaining authenticity. 2. Respect for Authenticity: While adaptation allows for experimentation, it's crucial to preserve the authenticity and integrity of the original cuisine. Maintaining the essential flavors, spices, and cooking methods pays homage to its roots. 3. Fusion with Local Ingredients: Introducing local ingredients into foreign dishes creates a unique fusion that marries two culinary worlds. It adds a fresh dimension while honoring both the original cuisine and the local produce. 4. Embracing Adaptability: Cultures are dynamic, and cuisines evolve with time. Embrace the adaptability of international cuisines, allowing for creative liberties that resonate with contemporary tastes while preserving the essence of tradition.

Infusing Diversity into Limited Ingredient Recipes

Limited ingredient recipes need not equate to limited flavors. Infusing diversity within these constraints is about strategic choices and inventive pairings. **1. Layering Flavors:** Each ingredient should contribute to multiple flavor profiles. For instance, herbs like basil or cilantro can add freshness and depth simultaneously. **2. Texture Play:** Manipulating textures can create an illusion of complexity. Crunchy nuts or crispy fried shallots can elevate a simple dish. **3. Utilizing Condiments and Sauces:** Leveraging condiments and sauces can be a game-changer. A well-made sauce or a carefully chosen condiment can transform a dish from mundane to extraordinary. **4. Ethnic Condiment Fusion:** Experiment by incorporating condiments from various cuisines. The tanginess of a Japanese ponzu sauce or the spiciness of a harissa can bring a whole new dimension to a dish, making it diverse and exciting.

Innovations in Fusion Cooking

Fusion cooking thrives on the amalgamation of diverse culinary traditions, paving the way for endless creative possibilities. **1. Unexpected Pairings:** Fusion cooking is all about breaking traditional boundaries by combining seemingly unrelated ingredients or techniques. Experiment with contrasting flavors and ingredients to discover unique and tantalizing combinations. **2.**

Blending Techniques: Merge cooking techniques from different cultures to create innovative dishes. For instance, combining French sous-vide with Asian stir-frying can yield remarkable results. **3. Cultural Exchange on the Plate:** Showcase the beauty of cultural exchange through food by presenting elements from different cuisines harmoniously on a single plate. This not only tantalizes taste buds but also celebrates diversity and unity through food. **4. Reviving Classics with a Twist:** Refreshing classic dishes by infusing them with elements from other cultures breathes new life into traditional recipes, making them more appealing to modern palates.

RISE AND SHINE: 5-INGREDIENT BREAKFAST INSPIRATIONS

Avocado Toast with Egg

Description of the Meal: Avocado toast with egg is a delicious and nutritious breakfast or brunch option. Creamy avocado pairs perfectly with a runny fried or poached egg, creating a satisfying and flavorful dish.

Ingredients:

- 2 slices of whole-grain bread
- 1 ripe avocado
- 2 eggs
- Salt and pepper to taste
- Optional toppings: red pepper flakes, sliced tomatoes, feta cheese

Instructions:

1. Toast the slices of whole-grain bread until golden brown.

2. While the bread is toasting, slice the avocado in half, remove the pit, and scoop the flesh into a bowl. Mash it with a fork and add a pinch of salt and pepper.

3. In a non-stick skillet, fry or poach the eggs according to your preference.

4. Spread the mashed avocado evenly onto the toasted bread slices.

5. Top each slice with a fried or poached egg.

6. Season with additional salt and pepper if desired. Add optional toppings like red pepper flakes, sliced tomatoes, or crumbled feta cheese.

7. Serve immediately and enjoy your flavorful avocado toast with egg!

Nutritional Information:

- *Calories:* Approximately 350-400 calories per serving (may vary based on specific ingredients and portion sizes).
- *Protein:* 15-20 grams
- *Fat:* 20-25 grams
- *Carbohydrates:* 30-35 grams

Greek Yogurt Parfait

Description of the Meal: A Greek yogurt parfait is a delightful combination of creamy yogurt, fresh fruits, crunchy granola, and a drizzle of honey, creating a balanced and satisfying breakfast or snack.

Ingredients:

- 1 cup Greek yogurt

- ½ cup granola
- ½ cup mixed fresh berries (strawberries, blueberries, raspberries)
- 2 tablespoons honey
- Optional toppings: sliced almonds, shredded coconut

Instructions:

1. In a glass or a bowl, start layering the ingredients. Begin with a spoonful of Greek yogurt at the bottom.

2. Add a layer of granola on top of the yogurt.

3. Follow with a layer of mixed fresh berries.

4. Repeat the layers until the glass or bowl is filled, ending with a final dollop of Greek yogurt on top.

5. Drizzle honey over the yogurt layer.

6. Garnish with optional toppings like sliced almonds or shredded coconut.

7. Serve immediately and enjoy the delightful flavors and textures of the Greek yogurt parfait!

Nutritional Information:

- *Calories:* Around 300-350 calories per serving (depending on the specific ingredients and amounts used).
- *Protein:* Approximately 15-20 grams
- *Fat:* 8-12 grams
- *Carbohydrates:* 40-45 grams

Banana-Oat Pancakes

Description of the Meal: Banana-oat pancakes are a healthier alternative to traditional pancakes, combining ripe bananas, oats, and eggs for a naturally sweet and nutritious breakfast option.

Ingredients:

- 2 ripe bananas
- 2 eggs
- ½ cup rolled oats
- ½ teaspoon baking powder
- ½ teaspoon vanilla extract
- Pinch of cinnamon (optional)
- Cooking oil or butter for frying

Instructions:

1. In a blender or food processor, combine the ripe bananas, eggs, rolled oats, baking powder, vanilla extract, and a pinch of cinnamon if desired. Blend until smooth.

2. Heat a non-stick skillet or griddle over medium heat and lightly grease it with cooking oil or butter.

3. Pour small amounts of the pancake batter onto the skillet to form pancakes.

4. Cook for 2-3 minutes on each side until golden brown.

5. Remove the pancakes from the skillet and repeat the process with the remaining batter.

6. Serve the banana-oat pancakes warm, topped

with fresh fruit, a drizzle of honey or maple syrup, and a sprinkle of additional oats if desired.

Nutritional Information:

- *Calories:* Approximately 250-300 calories per serving (based on ingredient quantities and toppings).
- *Protein:* 8-10 grams
- *Fat:* 8-10 grams
- *Carbohydrates:* 35-40 grams

Spinach and Feta Omelette

Description of the Meal: The spinach and feta omelette is a savory and nutritious breakfast option packed with protein, vitamins, and minerals. The combination of eggs, spinach, and feta cheese creates a flavorful dish.

Ingredients:

- 3 eggs
- 1 cup fresh spinach, chopped
- ¼ cup crumbled feta cheese
- Salt and pepper to taste
- Cooking oil or butter

Instructions:

1. Crack the eggs into a bowl, add salt, and whisk until well beaten.
2. Heat a non-stick skillet over medium heat and add a small amount of cooking oil or butter.
3. Pour the beaten eggs into the skillet and let them

    cook for a minute or until the edges begin to set.

4. Sprinkle chopped fresh spinach and crumbled feta cheese evenly over one side of the omelette.

5. Using a spatula, carefully fold the other half of the omelette over the filling.

6. Cook for another minute or until the cheese melts and the omelette is cooked to your desired doneness.

7. Slide the omelette onto a plate and season with pepper.

8. Serve the spinach and feta omelette hot, accompanied by a side of toast or fresh fruit.

Nutritional Information:

- *Calories:* Around 250-300 calories per serving (depending on the size of the eggs and cheese).
- *Protein:* Approximately 15-20 grams
- *Fat:* 15-18 grams
- *Carbohydrates:* 2-4 grams

Berry Smoothie Bowl

Description of the Meal: The berry smoothie bowl is a refreshing and nutritious breakfast option filled with the goodness of mixed berries, bananas, and various toppings, offering a burst of flavors and textures.

Ingredients:

- 1 cup mixed berries (strawberries, blueberries, raspberries)
- 1 ripe banana

- ½ cup Greek yogurt
- ¼ cup almond milk or any preferred milk
- Toppings: sliced fruits, granola, chia seeds, shredded coconut, honey

Instructions:

1. In a blender, combine the mixed berries, ripe banana, Greek yogurt, and almond milk. Blend until smooth and creamy.

2. Pour the berry smoothie into a bowl.

3. Top the smoothie with sliced fruits, granola, chia seeds, shredded coconut, a drizzle of honey, or any other preferred toppings.

4. Enjoy the berry smoothie bowl with a spoon, mixing the toppings into the smoothie as you eat.

Nutritional Information:

- *Calories:* Approximately 300-350 calories per serving (may vary based on the quantity of toppings and specific ingredients used).
- *Protein:* 10-15 grams
- *Fat:* 8-10 grams
- *Carbohydrates:* 40-45 grams

MIDDAY EATS MADE SIMPLE: 5-INGREDIENT LUNCH OPTIONS

Caprese Salad

Description of the Meal: Caprese salad is a refreshing and simple Italian dish that highlights fresh tomatoes, mozzarella cheese, basil leaves, olive oil, and balsamic vinegar. It's a perfect combination of flavors and textures.

Ingredients:

- 2 large tomatoes, sliced
- 8 oz fresh mozzarella cheese, sliced
- Fresh basil leaves
- 2 tablespoons extra-virgin olive oil
- 1 tablespoon balsamic vinegar
- Salt and pepper to taste

Instructions:

1. Arrange the tomato and mozzarella slices on a plate, alternating them.

2. Tuck basil leaves between the tomato and cheese slices.

3. Drizzle olive oil and balsamic vinegar over the salad.

4. Season with salt and pepper to taste.

5. Serve fresh and enjoy!

Nutritional Information: *(Per serving)*

- Calories: 250 kcal
- Fat: 18g
- Carbohydrates: 6g
- Protein: 14g

Veggie Quesadilla

Description of the Meal: Veggie quesadillas are a flavorful and versatile Mexican dish made with tortillas filled with a medley of sautéed vegetables, cheese, and spices, then toasted until crispy.

Ingredients:

- 4 large flour tortillas
- 1 cup shredded cheese (cheddar, Monterey Jack, or a blend)
- 1 bell pepper, thinly sliced
- 1 onion, thinly sliced
- 1 cup sliced mushrooms
- 1 cup spinach leaves
- 2 tablespoons olive oil
- Salt and pepper to taste
- Optional toppings: salsa, sour cream, guacamole

Instructions:

1. In a pan, heat olive oil over medium heat. Sauté the bell pepper, onion, mushrooms, and spinach until tender. Season with salt and pepper.

2. Place a tortilla on a flat surface. Spread a layer of shredded cheese on half of the tortilla.

3. Spoon the sautéed vegetable mixture over the cheese.

4. Fold the tortilla in half, covering the filling.

5. Repeat the process for the remaining tortillas.

6. Heat a pan over medium heat and place a filled tortilla in the pan. Cook until golden brown on both sides.

7. Repeat with the remaining quesadillas.

8. Slice each quesadilla into wedges and serve with optional toppings.

Nutritional Information: *(Per quesadilla)*

- Calories: 320 kcal
- Fat: 18g
- Carbohydrates: 30g
- Protein: 12g

Pesto Pasta

Description of the Meal: Pesto pasta is a classic Italian dish featuring pasta coated in a vibrant and flavorful sauce made with fresh basil, pine nuts, garlic, Parmesan cheese, and olive oil.

Ingredients:

- 12 oz pasta (such as spaghetti or penne)
- 2 cups fresh basil leaves

- ⅓ cup pine nuts
- 2 cloves garlic
- ½ cup grated Parmesan cheese
- ⅓ cup extra-virgin olive oil
- Salt and pepper to taste

Instructions:

1. Cook the pasta according to package instructions until al dente. Drain and set aside.

2. In a food processor, combine basil, pine nuts, garlic, and Parmesan cheese. Pulse until finely chopped.

3. While the processor is running, slowly add olive oil until the mixture forms a smooth paste. Season with salt and pepper.

4. Toss the cooked pasta with the pesto sauce until well coated.

5. Serve hot and garnish with extra Parmesan cheese if desired.

Nutritional Information: *(Per serving)*

- Calories: 480 kcal
- Fat: 26g
- Carbohydrates: 48g
- Protein: 12g

Tuna Salad Wraps

Description of the Meal: Tuna salad wraps are a light and satisfying option, combining canned tuna, crunchy vegetables, mayo, and spices, all wrapped in a tortilla for a convenient and tasty meal.

Ingredients:

- 2 cans (5 oz each) tuna, drained
- ½ cup mayonnaise
- 1 celery stalk, finely chopped
- 1 carrot, grated
- 2 tablespoons red onion, finely chopped
- 1 tablespoon lemon juice
- Salt and pepper to taste
- 4 large tortillas
- Lettuce leaves (optional)

Instructions:

1. In a bowl, mix together the tuna, mayonnaise, celery, carrot, red onion, lemon juice, salt, and pepper until well combined.

2. Lay out the tortillas and place lettuce leaves (if using) on each tortilla.

3. Spread the tuna salad mixture evenly over the lettuce leaves.

4. Roll up the tortillas tightly, enclosing the filling.

5. Cut each wrap in half diagonally and serve.

Nutritional Information: *(Per wrap)*

- Calories: 350 kcal
- Fat: 18g
- Carbohydrates: 25g

- Protein: 22g

Grilled Cheese and Tomato Soup

Description of the Meal: This comforting classic pairs a warm, creamy tomato soup with gooey grilled cheese sandwiches for a delightful and nostalgic meal.

Ingredients:

- 8 slices bread
- 8 oz cheddar cheese, sliced
- Butter for spreading
- 2 cans (14 oz each) tomato soup
- 1 cup milk
- Salt and pepper to taste

Instructions:

1. Heat a pan or griddle over medium heat.
2. Butter one side of each bread slice.
3. Place cheese slices between two slices of bread (buttered sides facing out).
4. Place the sandwiches on the heated pan and cook until golden brown on both sides and the cheese is melted.
5. In a pot, combine the tomato soup and milk. Heat over medium heat until warmed through.
6. Season the soup with salt and pepper to taste.
7. Serve the grilled cheese sandwiches alongside the tomato soup for dipping.

Nutritional Information: *(Per serving, 1 sandwich + soup)*

- Calories: 520 kcal
- Fat: 24g

- Carbohydrates: 52g
- Protein: 20g

Avocado Toast with Egg

Description of the Meal: Avocado toast with egg is a trendy and nutritious dish featuring mashed avocado on toasted bread, topped with a perfectly cooked egg, creating a satisfying breakfast or snack.

Ingredients:

- 4 slices whole-grain bread
- 2 ripe avocados
- 4 eggs
- Salt and pepper to taste
- Optional toppings: red pepper flakes, cherry tomatoes, feta cheese

Instructions:

1. Toast the slices of bread until golden brown.
2. In a bowl, mash the ripe avocados and season with salt and pepper.
3. Spread the mashed avocado evenly on each slice of toast.
4. Cook the eggs to your preference (fried, poached, or scrambled).
5. Place the cooked eggs on top of the avocado toast.
6. Add optional toppings if desired.
7. Serve immediately and enjoy!

Nutritional Information: *(Per serving, 1 slice)*

- Calories: 270 kcal
- Fat: 15g

- Carbohydrates: 26g
- Protein: 11g

DINNERTIME MAGIC: EFFORTLESS 5-INGREDIENT DINNERS

Caprese Chicken

Description of the meal: Caprese Chicken is a delightful dish inspired by the classic Italian Caprese salad. It combines the flavors of ripe tomatoes, fresh mozzarella cheese, basil, and balsamic glaze with juicy, tender chicken breasts.

Ingredients:

- 4 boneless, skinless chicken breasts
- 2 large tomatoes, sliced
- 8 ounces fresh mozzarella cheese, sliced
- Fresh basil leaves
- Balsamic glaze
- Salt and pepper to taste
- Olive oil

Instructions:

1. Preheat your oven to 400°F (200°C).

2. Season chicken breasts with salt and pepper.

3. Heat olive oil in an oven-safe skillet over medium-high heat.

4. Sear the chicken breasts for 3-4 minutes on each side until they get a golden brown color.

5. Top each chicken breast with tomato slices, mozzarella slices, and fresh basil leaves.

6. Transfer the skillet to the preheated oven and bake for 15-20 minutes or until the chicken is cooked through and the cheese is melted and bubbly.

7. Drizzle with balsamic glaze before serving.

Nutritional Information: *(Per Serving)*

- Calories: 320 kcal
- Protein: 42g
- Carbohydrates: 4g
- Fat: 15g
- Saturated Fat: 7g
- Cholesterol: 120mg
- Sodium: 380mg
- Fiber: 1g
- Sugar: 2g

Garlic Butter Shrimp

Description of the meal: Garlic Butter Shrimp is a quick and flavorful seafood dish that features succulent shrimp cooked in a rich, aromatic garlic butter sauce.

Ingredients:

- 1 pound large shrimp, peeled and deveined

- 4 cloves garlic, minced
- 4 tablespoons unsalted butter
- 2 tablespoons olive oil
- 2 tablespoons fresh parsley, chopped
- Red pepper flakes (optional)
- Salt and pepper to taste
- Lemon wedges for garnish

Instructions:

1. Heat olive oil and butter in a large skillet over medium heat.

2. Add minced garlic and red pepper flakes (if using) and sauté for about a minute until fragrant.

3. Add shrimp to the skillet and season with salt and pepper.

4. Cook the shrimp for 2-3 minutes on each side until they turn pink and opaque.

5. Sprinkle chopped parsley over the shrimp and toss to combine.

6. Serve the garlic butter shrimp hot with lemon wedges for a burst of citrus flavor.

Nutritional Information: *(Per Serving)*

- Calories: 280 kcal
- Protein: 24g
- Carbohydrates: 2g
- Fat: 19g
- Saturated Fat: 8g
- Cholesterol: 240mg
- Sodium: 400mg

- Fiber: 0g
- Sugar: 0g

Pesto Pasta

Description of the meal: Pesto Pasta is a simple yet flavorful dish that showcases al dente pasta tossed in a vibrant and herby basil pesto sauce.

Ingredients:

- 12 ounces pasta (such as spaghetti or penne)
- 2 cups fresh basil leaves
- ⅓ cup pine nuts or walnuts
- 2 cloves garlic, minced
- ½ cup grated Parmesan cheese
- ½ cup extra-virgin olive oil
- Salt and pepper to taste

Instructions:

1. Cook the pasta according to package instructions until it's al dente. Drain and set aside.

2. In a food processor, combine basil leaves, pine nuts (or walnuts), minced garlic, and Parmesan cheese. Pulse until finely chopped.

3. With the food processor running, gradually pour in the olive oil until the mixture forms a smooth paste. Season with salt and pepper.

4. Toss the cooked pasta with the prepared pesto sauce until well coated.

5. Serve the pesto pasta hot, garnished with additional grated Parmesan cheese if desired.

Nutritional Information: *(Per Serving)*

- Calories: 480 kcal
- Protein: 12g
- Carbohydrates: 42g
- Fat: 30g
- Saturated Fat: 5g
- Cholesterol: 10mg
- Sodium: 250mg
- Fiber: 3g
- Sugar: 2g

Honey Mustard Salmon

Description of the meal: Honey Mustard Salmon is a delectable dish that features tender salmon fillets glazed with a sweet and tangy honey mustard sauce.

Ingredients:

- 4 salmon fillets
- ¼ cup honey
- 2 tablespoons Dijon mustard
- 1 tablespoon whole-grain mustard
- 2 cloves garlic, minced
- 1 tablespoon olive oil
- Salt and pepper to taste
- Fresh dill for garnish (optional)

Instructions:

1. Preheat the oven to 400°F (200°C) and line a baking dish with parchment paper.

2. In a bowl, whisk together honey, Dijon mustard, whole-grain mustard, minced garlic, olive oil, salt, and pepper.

3. Place the salmon fillets in the prepared baking dish and brush the honey mustard mixture generously over each fillet.

4. Bake the salmon for 12-15 minutes or until it flakes easily with a fork and reaches your desired level of doneness.

5. Garnish with fresh dill before serving.

Nutritional Information: *(Per Serving)*

- Calories: 320 kcal
- Protein: 24g
- Carbohydrates: 14g
- Fat: 18g
- Saturated Fat: 3g
- Cholesterol: 65mg
- Sodium: 330mg
- Fiber: 0g
- Sugar: 14g

Taco Stuffed Peppers

Description of the meal: Taco Stuffed Peppers are a flavorful and colorful dish that combines the essence of tacos with the wholesome goodness of bell peppers stuffed with a savory filling.

Ingredients:

- 4 bell peppers (any color), halved and seeds removed
- 1 pound ground beef or turkey

- 1 cup cooked rice
- 1 cup black beans, drained and rinsed
- 1 cup corn kernels
- 1 packet taco seasoning
- 1 cup shredded cheddar cheese
- Fresh cilantro for garnish (optional)

Instructions:

1. Preheat the oven to 375°F (190°C) and prepare a baking dish.

2. In a skillet over medium heat, cook the ground beef or turkey until browned. Drain excess fat.

3. Add the cooked rice, black beans, corn, and taco seasoning to the skillet. Stir well to combine and cook for an additional 5 minutes.

4. Arrange the bell pepper halves in the baking dish and fill each pepper with the meat and rice mixture.

5. Top each stuffed pepper with shredded cheddar cheese.

6. Cover the dish with foil and bake for 25-30 minutes until the peppers are tender.

7. Garnish with fresh cilantro before serving.

Nutritional Information: *(Per Serving)*

- Calories: 380 kcal
- Protein: 25g
- Carbohydrates: 30g
- Fat: 18g
- Saturated Fat: 8g

- Cholesterol: 65mg
- Sodium: 800mg
- Fiber: 6g
- Sugar: 6g

Mushroom and Spinach Quesadillas

Description of the meal: Mushroom and Spinach Quesadillas are a delightful fusion of sautéed mushrooms, spinach, gooey cheese, and warm tortillas, creating a comforting and flavorful dish.

Ingredients:

- 8 small flour tortillas
- 2 cups sliced mushrooms
- 2 cups fresh spinach leaves
- 1 cup shredded mozzarella cheese
- 1 cup shredded cheddar cheese
- 2 tablespoons olive oil
- Salt and pepper to taste
- Salsa and sour cream for serving (optional)

Instructions:

1. Heat olive oil in a skillet over medium heat. Add sliced mushrooms and sauté until they're golden brown, about 5 minutes.

2. Add fresh spinach to the skillet and cook until wilted. Season with salt and pepper. Remove from heat.

3. Place a tortilla on a heated skillet or griddle over medium heat.

4. Sprinkle a layer of mozzarella and cheddar cheese

over half of the tortilla.

5. Spoon some of the mushroom and spinach mixture over the cheese.

6. Fold the tortilla in half to cover the filling and press gently with a spatula.

7. Cook for 2-3 minutes on each side until the tortilla turns golden brown and the cheese melts.

8. Repeat the process with the remaining tortillas and filling.

9. Cut the quesadillas into wedges and serve with salsa and sour cream if desired.

Nutritional Information: *(Per Serving, 2 quesadillas)*

- Calories: 480 kcal
- Protein: 20g
- Carbohydrates: 40g
- Fat: 26g
- Saturated Fat: 10g
- Cholesterol: 35mg
- Sodium: 800mg
- Fiber: 4g
- Sugar: 3g

SWEET SIMPLICITY: 5-INGREDIENT DESSERTS AND TREATS

No-Bake Peanut Butter Oatmeal Cookies

Description of the Meal: These No-Bake Peanut Butter Oatmeal Cookies are a delightful blend of creamy peanut butter, oats, and a touch of sweetness. Perfect for a quick, satisfying treat without the need for baking.

Ingredients:

- 1 cup creamy peanut butter
- 2 cups old-fashioned oats
- 1/2 cup honey or maple syrup
- 1/4 cup unsweetened cocoa powder
- 1/4 cup unsweetened shredded coconut (optional)
- 1 teaspoon vanilla extract

Instructions:

1. In a mixing bowl, combine peanut butter, oats, honey or maple syrup, cocoa powder, shredded coconut (if using), and vanilla extract. Stir until well combined.

2. Using a spoon or cookie scoop, portion out the mixture and shape it into cookie-sized rounds.

3. Place the cookies on a baking sheet lined with parchment paper.

4. Refrigerate for at least 30 minutes to allow the cookies to firm up.

5. Once set, enjoy your delicious No-Bake Peanut Butter Oatmeal Cookies!

Nutritional Information: (Per Serving)

- Calories: 180 kcal
- Carbohydrates: 20g
- Protein: 5g
- Fat: 10g
- Fiber: 3g

Strawberry Frozen Yogurt

Description of the Meal: This Strawberry Frozen Yogurt is a refreshing and creamy dessert that's bursting with fruity flavor. It's a simple and healthy treat made with fresh strawberries and yogurt.

Ingredients:

- 3 cups frozen strawberries
- 2 cups Greek yogurt
- 1/4 cup honey or agave syrup (adjust to taste)
- 1 teaspoon vanilla extract

Instructions:

1. In a blender or food processor, add frozen strawberries, Greek yogurt, honey or agave syrup,

and vanilla extract.

2. Blend the ingredients until smooth and creamy.

3. Taste the mixture and adjust sweetness if needed by adding more honey or syrup.

4. Transfer the mixture into a freezer-safe container and freeze for 4-6 hours or until firm.

5. Once frozen, scoop out the Strawberry Frozen Yogurt and serve chilled.

Nutritional Information: (Per Serving)

- Calories: 120 kcal
- Carbohydrates: 20g
- Protein: 7g
- Fat: 1g
- Fiber: 3g

Chocolate Avocado Mousse

Description of the Meal: This Chocolate Avocado Mousse is a rich, velvety dessert that combines the goodness of avocados with the indulgence of chocolate. It's a healthier alternative to traditional mousse recipes.

Ingredients:

- 2 ripe avocados
- 1/3 cup cocoa powder
- 1/4 cup honey or maple syrup (adjust to taste)
- 1 teaspoon vanilla extract
- Pinch of salt
- Optional toppings: sliced strawberries, shaved chocolate

Instructions:

1. Cut the avocados in half, remove the pits, and scoop the flesh into a blender or food processor.
2. Add cocoa powder, honey or maple syrup, vanilla extract, and a pinch of salt to the blender.
3. Blend the ingredients until smooth and creamy, scraping down the sides as needed.
4. Taste the mousse and adjust sweetness if desired.
5. Divide the mousse into serving cups or bowls.
6. Chill in the refrigerator for at least 30 minutes before serving.
7. Garnish with sliced strawberries or shaved chocolate if desired.

Nutritional Information: (Per Serving)

- Calories: 180 kcal
- Carbohydrates: 18g
- Protein: 3g
- Fat: 12g
- Fiber: 7g

Coconut Macaroons

Description of the Meal: These Coconut Macaroons are sweet, chewy, and packed with coconut flavor. They are simple to make and perfect for anyone with a sweet tooth craving a delightful treat.

Ingredients:

- 3 cups shredded coconut (sweetened or unsweetened)

- 1/2 cup sweetened condensed milk
- 2 egg whites
- 1 teaspoon vanilla extract
- Pinch of salt

Instructions:

1. Preheat your oven to 325°F (160°C). Line a baking sheet with parchment paper.

2. In a mixing bowl, combine shredded coconut, sweetened condensed milk, vanilla extract, and a pinch of salt.

3. In a separate clean bowl, whisk the egg whites until they form stiff peaks.

4. Gently fold the whipped egg whites into the coconut mixture until well combined.

5. Using a spoon or cookie scoop, form mounds of the mixture onto the prepared baking sheet, leaving space between each mound.

6. Bake for 20-25 minutes or until the macaroons turn golden brown around the edges.

7. Remove from the oven and let them cool completely on the baking sheet before serving.

Nutritional Information: (Per Serving)

- Calories: 120 kcal
- Carbohydrates: 10g
- Protein: 2g
- Fat: 8g
- Fiber: 2g

SEASONAL SPECIALS: 5-INGREDIENT RECIPES FOR FESTIVITIES

Stuffed Mushroom Caps

Description of the Meal: Stuffed Mushroom Caps are savory appetizers filled with a delightful mixture of breadcrumbs, cheese, herbs, and mushrooms, baked to perfection.

Ingredients:

- 12 large mushroom caps
- 1 cup breadcrumbs
- 1/2 cup grated Parmesan cheese
- 1/4 cup chopped parsley
- 2 cloves garlic, minced
- 2 tablespoons olive oil
- Salt and pepper to taste

Instructions:

1. Preheat the oven to 375°F (190°C). Clean the mushroom caps and remove the stems.

2. In a mixing bowl, combine breadcrumbs, Parmesan cheese, parsley, garlic, olive oil, salt, and pepper.

3. Stuff each mushroom cap generously with the breadcrumb mixture, pressing gently to pack it in.

4. Place the stuffed mushroom caps on a baking sheet lined with parchment paper.

5. Bake for 18-20 minutes or until the mushrooms are tender and the tops are golden brown.

6. Serve hot and enjoy this delicious appetizer.

Nutritional Information: *(per serving)*

- Calories: 120kcal
- Fat: 6g
- Carbohydrates: 12g
- Protein: 5g

Cranberry Brie Bites

Description of the Meal: Cranberry Brie Bites are delightful appetizers featuring the creamy goodness of Brie cheese paired with sweet cranberry sauce, all nestled in crispy phyllo pastry cups.

Ingredients:

- 24 mini phyllo pastry cups
- 6 oz Brie cheese, cut into small cubes
- 1/2 cup cranberry sauce
- Fresh rosemary sprigs (for garnish)

Instructions:

1. Preheat the oven to 350°F (175°C). Place the phyllo pastry cups on a baking sheet.

2. Add a cube of Brie cheese into each pastry cup.

3. Top the Brie with a small spoonful of cranberry sauce.

4. Bake in the preheated oven for 5-7 minutes, or until the Brie is melted and the edges of the pastry cups are golden brown.

5. Garnish with fresh rosemary sprigs and serve warm.

Nutritional Information: *(per serving)*

- Calories: 60kcal
- Fat: 3g
- Carbohydrates: 6g
- Protein: 2g

Pesto Pasta Salad

Description of the Meal: Pesto Pasta Salad is a vibrant and flavorful dish made with pasta tossed in a basil pesto sauce, combined with cherry tomatoes, fresh mozzarella, and pine nuts.

Ingredients:

- 8 oz pasta (such as fusilli or penne)
- 1/2 cup basil pesto
- 1 cup cherry tomatoes, halved
- 1 cup fresh mozzarella balls, halved
- 1/4 cup pine nuts, toasted

- Fresh basil leaves for garnish
- Salt and pepper to taste

Instructions:

1. Cook the pasta according to package instructions until al dente. Drain and rinse under cold water.

2. In a large mixing bowl, combine the cooked pasta, basil pesto, cherry tomatoes, fresh mozzarella, and toasted pine nuts. Toss gently until well combined.

3. Season with salt and pepper to taste.

4. Garnish with fresh basil leaves.

5. Serve chilled or at room temperature.

Nutritional Information: *(per serving)*

- Calories: 380kcal
- Fat: 22g
- Carbohydrates: 32g
- Protein: 14g

Prosciutto-Wrapped Asparagus

Description of the Meal: Prosciutto-Wrapped Asparagus is an elegant appetizer where tender asparagus spears are wrapped in salty prosciutto and baked until crispy.

Ingredients:

- 24 asparagus spears, tough ends trimmed
- 12 slices prosciutto, halved lengthwise
- 2 tablespoons olive oil
- Salt and black pepper to taste

Instructions:

1. Preheat the oven to 400°F (200°C). Line a baking sheet with parchment paper.

2. Toss the asparagus spears with olive oil, salt, and pepper.

3. Bundle 2 asparagus spears together and wrap with a piece of prosciutto, starting from the bottom and spiraling to the top.

4. Place the wrapped asparagus on the prepared baking sheet.

5. Bake for 10-12 minutes or until the asparagus is tender and the prosciutto is crispy.

6. Serve immediately as a delightful appetizer.

Nutritional Information: *(per serving)*

- Calories: 90kcal
- Fat: 6g
- Carbohydrates: 2g
- Protein: 7g

CRAFTING CULINARY MEMORIES WITH 5 INGREDIENTS

Reflecting on Experiences and Creativity of 5 Ingredients Cooking

In the realm of culinary arts, the concept of 5 ingredients cooking has gained momentum, capturing the essence of simplicity while fostering creativity. This minimalist approach to cooking involves crafting flavorful dishes using only five key components. It's a delightful intersection of culinary finesse and innovative simplicity, encouraging both novice and seasoned cooks to explore and create.

Embracing Limited Ingredients

The essence of 5 ingredients cooking lies in its limitation.

Restricting oneself to only five ingredients sounds confining initially, but it paradoxically opens up a world of possibilities. This constraint sparks creativity, challenging individuals to innovate within the bounds of simplicity. By focusing on a handful of elements, one must delve deeper into their flavors, textures, and interactions. Each ingredient carries weight and significance, demanding thoughtful consideration and utilization in inventive ways.

Creativity Unleashed through Constraints

Contrary to popular belief, limitations often breed innovation. In the context of cooking with five ingredients, this limitation serves as a catalyst for creativity. Chefs and home cooks alike are forced to think outside the box, experimenting with unexpected combinations and techniques to achieve a harmonious balance of flavors and textures. The challenge of making a dish shine with a concise ingredient list pushes individuals to explore their culinary ingenuity, resulting in surprising and delightful outcomes.

Nurturing Culinary Innovation

The realm of 5 ingredients cooking isn't solely about the outcome on the plate; it's also about the journey. It nurtures culinary innovation by encouraging individuals to rely on their intuition, improvisation skills, and understanding of ingredient synergy. This style of cooking fosters a deeper connection between the cook and their creations, allowing for a more intimate and explorative culinary experience.

Heightened Focus on Ingredient Quality

With a limited ingredient list, each component assumes paramount importance. There's an increased emphasis on the quality of ingredients rather than their quantity. Chefs and cooks need to select top-notch, fresh produce or premium ingredients to elevate the dish. This emphasis on quality not only enhances the final outcome but also encourages mindfulness about sourcing and utilizing ingredients sustainably.

Culinary Education and Experimentation

5 ingredients cooking serves as an excellent platform for culinary education and experimentation. It's a canvas for honing skills, understanding flavor profiles, and exploring the intricacies of ingredients. This style of cooking is inclusive, inviting amateurs to explore the culinary landscape without feeling overwhelmed. It's a journey of learning through hands-on experiences, where mistakes are welcomed as stepping stones toward mastery.

Encouraging Reader's Culinary Adventures

Culinary exploration is an enriching journey that transcends mere sustenance. Encouraging readers to embark on their own culinary adventures is akin to igniting a spark of passion and creativity within them. It's an invitation to explore diverse cuisines, experiment with flavors, and foster a deeper appreciation for the art of cooking.

Inviting Exploration Beyond Comfort Zones

Encouraging readers to delve into culinary adventures entails nudging them beyond their comfort zones. It involves introducing them to new ingredients, techniques, or cuisines they might not have previously considered. It's about broadening horizons and embracing the unknown, fostering a sense of curiosity and excitement about the vast world of food.

Providing Practical Guidance

While embarking on culinary adventures, readers often seek guidance. Providing practical tips, step-by-step instructions, and insights into various cooking methods empowers individuals to navigate uncharted culinary territories confidently. Recipes, tutorials, and explanations of fundamental cooking techniques serve as valuable resources in their culinary explorations.

Celebrating Cultural Diversity through Food

Food serves as a gateway to understanding and celebrating diverse cultures. Encouraging culinary adventures involves highlighting the richness of different cuisines, shedding light on their histories, traditions, and unique flavor profiles. By embracing foods from various cultures, readers not only expand their culinary repertoire but also foster a deeper appreciation for cultural diversity.

Fostering Confidence and Creativity

Empowering readers to embark on culinary adventures is also about nurturing their confidence and creativity in the kitchen. Encouraging experimentation, improvisation, and adaptation within recipes instills a sense of ownership and creativity in cooking. It's about fostering a mindset where mistakes are valuable learning experiences, and culinary success is defined by the joy of exploration and creation.

Community Engagement and Sharing Experiences

Encouraging culinary adventures extends beyond individual journeys; it encompasses building a community of enthusiastic cooks. Platforms that facilitate sharing experiences, exchanging recipes, and engaging in conversations about culinary discoveries create a sense of camaraderie. This community-driven approach fosters an environment where everyone feels supported and inspired to continue their culinary explorations.

CONCLUSION

Recapitulation of the 5-Ingredient Cooking Journey

In our culinary expedition centered around the concept of 5-ingredient cooking, we've traversed a realm where simplicity harmonizes with flavor, and efficiency intertwines with creativity. This journey celebrates the elegance of minimalism, emphasizing five core ingredients to craft delightful meals. Each dish, a testament to the synergy of simplicity and taste, inviting both seasoned chefs and novice cooks to embark on a flavorful adventure.

1. Embracing Simplicity: The essence of 5-ingredient cooking lies in its simplicity. By limiting ingredients to five, we've unlocked a world of culinary possibilities without overwhelming complexity. This approach emphasizes quality over quantity, urging us to harness the potential of a few essential elements to create gastronomic marvels.

2. Unleashing Creativity: Constraints often fuel creativity, and in the realm of 5-ingredient cooking, this is palpable. Within the confines of five ingredients, innovation blossoms. Experimentation flourishes as cooks explore various combinations, substitutions, and techniques to craft unique flavors and textures.

3. Amplifying Flavor Dynamics: The restricted ingredient palette in 5-ingredient cooking is not limiting; instead, it amplifies the significance of each component. Every ingredient plays a pivotal role, contributing distinct flavors, textures, and aromas that harmonize to create a symphony on the palate.

4. Streamlining Culinary Efficiency: Efficiency reigns supreme in the 5-ingredient paradigm. This approach streamlines meal preparation, reducing shopping lists, cooking time, and cleanup efforts. It appeals to individuals seeking convenient yet scrumptious culinary experiences without compromising on taste or quality.

5. Cultivating Confidence: Beyond the kitchen, 5-ingredient cooking fosters culinary confidence. It encourages experimentation and empowers individuals to trust their instincts while exploring flavors. This confidence extends beyond the realm of cooking, influencing problem-solving and creative thinking in diverse aspects of life.

As we look back on this expedition through the lens of 5-ingredient cooking, we witness the marriage of simplicity and innovation, taste and efficiency. It's not merely about the dishes we've crafted but the journey itself—the lessons learned, the creativity sparked, and the culinary confidence instilled.

Encouraging Readers to Explore and Innovate

Embarking on a culinary journey is not solely about following recipes; it's an invitation to explore, experiment, and innovate. Here, we urge readers to step beyond the confines of traditional cooking and embrace their inner culinary adventurers.

1. Embrace Curiosity: The heart of culinary exploration lies in curiosity. Encouraging readers to ask questions, try unconventional ingredient pairings, and explore diverse cuisines fosters a sense of discovery. Curiosity fuels innovation and leads to the creation of novel, enticing flavors.

2. Experiment with Ingredients: Experimentation is the cornerstone of culinary innovation. Encourage readers to step out of their comfort zones by experimenting with unfamiliar ingredients or tweaking traditional recipes. It's through these experiments that unexpected flavors and textures often emerge.

3. Foster a Fearless Attitude: Fear of failure can hinder culinary exploration. Advocate for a fearless attitude towards cooking—mistakes are part of the journey, often leading to unforeseen culinary masterpieces. Encourage readers to embrace mishaps as learning opportunities.

4. Emphasize Personal Touch: Cooking is an art, and like any art form, it thrives on personal expression. Encourage readers to infuse their dishes with their unique flair, whether through presentation, seasoning, or creative plating techniques. This personal touch adds depth and character to culinary creations.

5. Promote Sharing and Learning: Encourage readers to share their culinary experiments, successes, and failures with others. Engaging in a community that celebrates learning and sharing experiences fosters a culture of continuous improvement and inspiration.

By inspiring readers to embark on their own culinary expeditions, embracing curiosity, experimentation, and fearlessness, we catalyze a journey of endless possibilities in the kitchen.